Titan Training: 100 Elite Gym Workouts

By: Fred Hughes

I am dedicated to serving the public and helping others achieve their physical or mental goals. I believe that fitness is one of the core components for living a successful life. I have spent the last 10 years formulating and testing fitness regiments. With 5 years in the United States Marine Corps Infantry, 2 years of Diplomatic Security overseas, and certifications in both Personal Training and High Intensity Training, my programs are proven to increase athletic performance.

This program is designed for those aspiring a higher level athletic performance or those serving this great nation who require annual fitness tests. The workouts involve prior knowledge of common exercises and should not be attempted by those uncomfortable with gym equipment. These workouts are not easy and will require a dedication and willingness to believe in one's inner self. Life is about choices. The choice to become physically and mentally fit is within everyone.

As Babe Ruth once said, "It's hard to beat a person who never gives up."

Waiver of Liability

By purchasing, viewing, or using this workout program or the workouts within, you are waiving any liability to Fred Hughes or any other sources affiliated with this publication. Injuries may occur in any workout program and can occur in the workouts and exercises listed in this publication. Always consult a physician before starting any physical fitness program or new fitness routine.

<u>Workout 1:</u>

3 Sets of 8-10 Reps Incline Bench Press
Wt.________________
3 Sets of 8-10 Reps Cable Chest Fly or Seated Machine
Fly
Wt.________________
3 Sets of 8-10 Reps Decline Dumbbell Bench Press
Wt.________________

2 Rounds for Time (Abs):
20 Russian Core Twists
20 Bicycle Crunches
20 Laying Leg Lifts
20 Ball Crunches
Time: ______________

2 Rounds for Time:
10 Barbell Bench Press
20 Push-ups
30 Second Abs Plank
10 Bench Dips
30 Crunches
Time: ______________

Cardio:
10 Sets of 30 Seconds of Running / 30 Seconds Rest
(Treadmill Incline level 12, Pace 8-10 or 6-8 min Mile)
Sets Completed: __ __ __ __ __ __ __ __ __ __

<u>Workout 2:</u>

3 Sets of 8-10 Reps Seated Leg Ext. (Machine)
Wt.______________
3 Sets of 8-10 Reps Seated Machine Calf Raises
Wt.______________
3 Sets of 8-10 Reps Seated Leg Curl (Machine)
Wt.______________
3 Sets of 8-10 Reps Seated Leg Press
Wt.______________
3 Sets of 8-10 Reps Barbell Squats
Wt.______________

2 Rounds for Time:
20 Walking Lunges (10 Each Leg)
30 Crunches
10 Jumping Air Squats
30 Russian Twists
30 Jumping Jacks
Time: _____________

Cardio:
20 Min. on Elliptical maintaining HR between 145-165
Distance: _____________

<u>Workout 3:</u>

3 Sets of 8-10 Reps Cable Lat Pull Downs
Wt._______________
3 Sets of 8-10 Reps of Pull Ups
Wt._______________
3 Sets of 8-10 Reps Machine Back Fly
Wt._______________
3 Sets of 8-10 Seated Cable Machine Rows
Wt._______________

2 Rounds for Time:
20 Bent Over Dumbbell Rows (10 Each Arm)
20 Pushups
20 Dumbbell Shrugs
20 Laying Leg Lifts
Time: _______________

Cardio:
1000m on the Rowing Machine or 20 Minutes on Stair Climber

<u>Workout 4:</u>

3 Sets of 8-10 Reps Seated Overhead Dumbbell Press
Wt.________________
3 Sets of 8-10 Reps Barbell Upright Rows
Wt.________________
3 Sets of 8-10 Reps Seated Bent Over Rear Deltoid
Raise
Wt.________________

2 Rounds for Time:
15 DB Front Raise
15 DB Side Raise
15 DB 45 Degree Raise
Time: ______________

Cardio:
Biking Pyramid 1-10-1
Stay at each level of resistance for 1 minute increasing to
level 10 then decrease back to level 1 (Bike level 1 for 1
minute, then level 2 for one minute, then 3 for one
minute- all the way to 10 and then back down to 1).
Attempt to maintain 100rpm at each level.
Distance: ______________

<u>Workout 5:</u>

3 Sets of 8-10 Reps Cable Bicep Curls
Wt._______________
3 Sets of 8-10 Reps Cable Tri Extensions
Wt._______________
3 Sets of 8-10 Reps Machine Curls
Wt._______________
3 Sets of 8-10 Reps Machine Triceps
Wt._______________

2 Rounds for Time:
10 Dumbbell Hammer Curls (each arm)
10 Bench Dips
10 Dumbbell Curls (each arm)
10 Barbell Skull Crushers
Time: _______________

2 Rounds for Time:
20 Ball Crunches
20 Hanging Knee Raises
20 Russian Twists
20 Flutter Kicks
Time: _______________

<u>Workout 6:</u>

Max Repetitions (1 Minute Break Between Workouts)
2 Minutes of Mountain Climbers
Reps ______________
2 Minutes of Ball Crunches
Reps ______________
2 Minutes of Jumping Jacks
Reps ______________
2 Minutes of Side-to-Side Hops
Reps ______________

Then: 3-Mile Slow Jog (Level 5-6 or 10-11 Minute
Miles) Incline #4
Time: ______________

<u>Workout 7:</u>

3 Sets of 8-10 Reps Barbell Bench Press
Wt.________________
3 Sets of 8-10 Reps Military Overhead Press
Wt.________________
3 Sets of 8-10 Reps Cable Triceps Extension
Wt.________________

2 Rounds for Time:
10 Dips
20 Push Ups
10 Dumbbell Front Raise
20 Decline Push Ups
10 Overhead Dumbbell Triceps Extensions
Time: ________________

Cardio:
2 X ½ mile at 4:00min each ½ mile. Target Pace set as 8-minute mile on Treadmill (60 Sec Rest Between each ½ Mile) Sets Completed: __ __
4 X ¼ Mile at 2:00min each ¼ mile. Target Pace set as 8-minute mile pace on Treadmill (60 Sec Rest Between each 1/4 mile) Sets Completed: __ __ __ __
4 X 1/8 Mile at 45 seconds. Target pace set as 6-Minute Mile on Treadmill (30 Sec Rest Between Rounds) Sets Completed: __ __ __ __

<u>Workout 8:</u>

3 Sets of 8-10 Reps Machine Leg Extensions
Wt._______________
3 Sets of 8-10 Reps Machine Leg Curls
Wt._______________
3 Sets of 8-10 Reps Machine Calf Raises
Wt._______________
3 Sets of 8-10 Reps Machine Leg Press
Wt._______________

2 Rounds for Time:
20 1 and ¼ air squats
20 Jumping Lunges
20 Air Calf Raises
30 Jumping Jacks
Time: _______________

Cardio:
20 Minutes of Stair Climber (Stair Master)
1000 Meter Row
Time: _______________

<u>Workout 9:</u>

3 Sets of 8-10 Reps Cable Lat Pull Down
Wt._________________
3 Sets of 8-10 Reps Machine Curls
Wt._________________
3 Sets of 8-10 Reps Machine Tri
Wt._________________
3 Sets of 8-10 Pull Ups
Wt._________________

2 Rounds for Time:
15 Cable Tri Extensions
15 Cable Bicep Cable Curls
15 Cable Face Pulls
15 Dips
Time: _____________

Cardio:
1.5 Mile Sprint at Level 8-10 (Between 6:00-8:00 minute
mile pace)
Time: _____________

<u>Workout 10:</u>

Cardio Day

Biking Pyramid 1-10-1
Stay at each level of resistance for 1 minute increasing to level 10 then decrease back to level 1 (Bike level 1 for 1 minute, then level 2 for one minute, then 3 for one minute- all the way to 10 and then back down to 1). Attempt to maintain 100rpm at each level.
Distance: _____________

Then: 10 Sets of 30 Seconds of Running / 30 Seconds Rest (Incline level 12, Pace 8-10 or 6-8 min Mile) Sets Completed: __ __ __ __ __ __ __ __ __ __

Finish with 15 Minutes of Stair Climber

<u>Workout 11:</u>

3 Sets of 8-10 Reps Barbell Close Grip Bench Press
Wt._______________
3 Sets of 8-10 Reps Incline Dumbbell Bench Press
Wt._______________
3 Sets of 8-10 Reps Seated Dumbbell Overhead Press
Wt._______________
3 Sets of 8-10 Reps Dips (Scaled Bench or Assisted
Machine)
Wt._______________

2 Rounds for Time:
10 Standing Cable Fly Angled Down
10 Standing Cable Tri Extensions
10 Standing Cable Fly Angled Up
10 Standing Cable Chest Press
Time: _______________

Cardio:
20 Min of Elliptical Machine HR 145-165 or sub 6 min
per mile pace
Distance: _______________

<u>Workout 12:</u>

3 Sets of 8-10 Reps Barbell Squats
Wt._________________
3 Sets of 8-10 Reps (Per Leg) Walking Dumbbell
Lunges
Wt._______________
3 Sets of 8-10 Reps of Barbell Romanian Deadlift
Wt._______________
3 Sets of 8-10 Reps Machine Calf Raise
Wt._______________

2 Rounds for Time:
20 Russian Twists
20 Hanging Knee Raise
20 Crunches
30 Sec Plank Left Side
30 Sec Plank Right Side
Time: ______________

Cardio:
30 Minutes of Bike (Medium Level/ Maintain RPM 100)
Level: ______________

<u>Workout 13:</u>

3 Sets of 8-10 Reps Pull Ups (Machine Assisted if needed)
Wt.______________
3 Sets of 8-10 Reps Barbell Bent over Rows
Wt.______________
3 Sets of 8-10 Reps Cable Face Pull
Wt.______________
3 Sets of 8-10 Reps Machine Back Fly
Wt.______________

2 Rounds for Time:
10 Dumbbell Bicep Curls
20 Dumbbell Shrugs
10 Dumbbell Hammer Curls
20 Dumbbell Shrugs
Time: ______________

Light Cardio:
10 Minutes on the Elliptical
Distance: ______________

<u>Workout 14:</u>

3 Sets of 8-10 Reps of DB Bench Press
Wt.________________
3 Sets of 8-10 Reps Cable Tri Extension
Wt.________________
3 Sets of 8-10 Reps of Laying DB Chest Fly
Wt.________________
3 Sets of 8-10 Reps Overhead DB Press
Wt.________________

2 Rounds for Time:
15 DB Front Raise
15 Push Ups
15 DB Side Raise
15 Push Ups
15 DB 45* Raise
Time: ________________

Cardio:
Biking Pyramid 1-10-1
Stay at each level of resistance for 1 minute increasing to level 10 then decrease back to level 1 (Bike level 1 for 1 minute, then level 2 for one minute, then level 3 for one minute- all the way to 10 and then back down to 1).
Attempt to maintain 100rpm at each level.
Distance: ________________

<u>Workout 15:</u>

3 Sets of 8-10 Reps of Leg Extensions
Wt._________________
3 Sets of 8-10 Reps Leg Curls
Wt._________________
3 Sets of 8-10 Reps Machine Leg Press
Wt._________________
3 Sets of 8-10 Reps of Machine Calf Raise
Wt._________________

2 Rounds for Time:
20 1 and ¼ Air Squats
20 Crunches
20 Bodyweight Lunges (10 Each Leg)
20 Russian Twists
20 Jumping Jacks
Time: _______________

Cardio:
2X 1 Mile Sprints (Level 8-10 or 6:00-8:00 Min Pace) –
60 Sec rest between miles
Time: _______________ _______________

<u>Workout 16:</u>

3 Sets of 8-10 Reps Seated Cable Rows
Wt.________________
3 Sets of 8-10 Reps Cable Face Pulls
Wt.________________
3 Sets of 8-10 Reps Cable Lat Pull Down
Wt.________________
3 Sets of 8-10 Reps Cable Straight Bar Bicep Curls
Wt.________________

2 Rounds for Time:
10 DB Hammer Curls
10 Pull Ups
30 Hanging Knee Raises
10 DB 1 and ¼ Curls
10 Push Ups
Time: ______________

Cardio:
20 Minutes of Speed Walking on Treadmill at #12
Incline
Distance: ____________

<u>Workout 17:</u>

3 Sets of 8-10 Reps Barbell Decline Bench Press
Wt.________________
3 Sets of 8-10 Reps Machine Chest Fly
Wt.________________
3 Sets of 8-10 Reps Barbell Incline Bench Press
Wt.________________
3 Sets of 8-10 Reps Dumbbell Laying Close Grip Bench Press
Wt.________________

2 Rounds for Time:
20 Incline Push Ups
20 Russian Twists
20 Push Ups
20 Crunches
20 Bicycle Crunches
Time: ________________

Cardio:
10 Sets of 30 Seconds of Running / 15 Seconds Rest
(Incline level 12, Pace 8-10 or 6-8 min Mile)
Sets Completed: __ __ __ __ __ __ __ __ __ __

<u>Workout 18:</u>

3 Sets of 8-10 Reps Barbell Front Squats
Wt.________________
3 Sets of 8-10 Reps Leg Ext (2 Sec Hold at Top)
Wt.________________
3 Sets of 8-10 Reps Leg Curl (2 Sec Hold at Top)
Wt.________________
3 Sets of 8-10 Reps Machine Leg Press
Wt.________________

2 Rounds for Time:
20 Air Squats
20 Crunches
20 Walking Lunges (10 Each Leg)
20 Laying Leg Lifts
20 Bunny Hops (Jumping up and down landing on toes
focusing on calf muscles)
Time: ______________

Cardio:
20 Minutes of Running at Level 6 (10 Min Pace but
Incline #12)
Distance: ______________

<u>Workout 19:</u>

3 Sets of 8-10 Reps Dumbbell Bent over Rows (per arm)
Wt._______________
3 Sets of 8-10 Reps Cable Lat Pull Down
Wt._______________
3 Sets of 8-10 Reps Machine Back Fly
Wt._______________
3 Sets of 8-10 Reps Pull Ups
Wt._______________

2 Rounds for Time:
20 Flutter Kicks
20 Laying Superman
20 Crunches
20 Good Mornings (Standing Hip Hinge)
Time: _______________

Cardio:
Run-
2 X 1/2mile at 4:00min pace (60 Sec Rest Between ½ Miles)
2 X ¼ Mile at 2:00min pace (30 Sec Rest Between 1/4 miles)
4 X 1/8mile at :45 second pace (30 Sec Rest Between Rounds)
Sets Completed: __ __ __ __ __ __ __ __

<u>Workout 20:</u>

3 Sets of 8-10 Reps Military Barbell Press
Wt.________________
3 Sets of 8-10 Reps Barbell Shrugs
Wt.________________
3 Sets of 8-10 Reps Cable Face Pulls
Wt.________________
3 Sets of 8-10 Reps Seated Dumbbell Side (lateral) Raise
Wt.________________

2 Rounds for Time:
20 Small Arm Circles Forward
20 Overhead Air Press
20 Small Arm Circles Backward
20 Overhead Air Press
20 Large Arm Circles Forward
20 Large Arm Circles Backward
20 Russian Twists
Time: ______________

Cardio:
20 Minutes of Stair Climber at Medium Speed
500-Meter Row
Time: ______________

<u>Workout 21:</u>

3 Sets of 8-10 Reps Cable 1 Arm Bicep Curls (per arm)
Wt.______________
3 Sets of 8-10 Reps Cable 1 Arm Tri Ext (per arm)
Wt.______________
3 Sets of 8-10 Reps Dumbbell Hammer Curls
Wt.______________
3 Sets of 8-10 Reps Overhead Dumbbell Tri Extension
Wt.______________

2 Rounds for Time:
(21 Gun)
7 Half the way up Barbell Curls
Then: 7 Barbell Curls from 90* position to up position
Then: 7 Complete Barbell Curls
Time: ______________

After Superset:
40 Diamond Push Ups

Cardio:
20-Minute Elliptical at HR 145-165 (Sub 6 Minute Pace)
Distance: ____________

<u>Workout 22:</u>

Cardio Day:
1 Mile Run at Slow Pace (10:00-11:00 Minute Pace)
Time: _______________
500 Meters on Rowing Machine
Time: _______________
1 Mile Run at Moderate Pace (8:00-10:00 Minute Pace)
Time: _______________
500 Meters on Rowing Machine
Time: _______________
1 Mile Run at Fast Pace (6:00-8:00 Minute Pace)
Time: _______________
500 Meters on Rowing Machine
Time: _______________

<u>Workout 23</u>:

3 Sets of 8-10 Reps 1 and ¼ Barbell Bench Press
Wt.________________
3 Sets of 8-10 Reps Machine Chest Fly
Wt.________________
3 Sets of 8-10 Reps Barbell Incline Bench Press
Wt.________________
3 Sets of 8-10 Reps Dumbbell Decline Bench Press (2 Sec Hold at Top)
Wt.________________

2 Rounds for Time:
10 Standing Med Ball Press
20 Russian Twists
10 Laying Med Ball Press/Throw Catch
20 Crunches
Time: ________________

Cardio:
5-Mile Bike Ride at Sub 6 Minute Pace
Time: ________________

<u>Workout 24:</u>

2 Rounds for Time:
20 Jumping Air Squats
20 Russian Twists
20 Jumping Lunges
20 Laying Leg Lifts
Time: _______________

3 Sets of 8-10 Reps Machine Leg Extensions (2 Sec Hold at Top and 4 Count Back Down)
Wt._______________
3 Sets of 8-10 Reps Machine Leg Curls (2 Sec Hold at Top and 4 Count Back Down)
Wt._______________
3 Sets of 8-10 Reps Machine Calf Raise (2 Sec Hold at Top)
Wt._______________
3 Sets of 8-10 Reps Machine Leg Press
Wt._______________

Cardio:
2000-Meter Row on Rowing Machine
Time: _______________
100 Jumping Jacks
Time: _______________

<u>Workout 25</u>:

Pull/Push/Sit-up Pyramid

1-10-1 of Pull Ups (1,2,3,4,5,6,7,8,9,10,9,8,7,6,5,4,3,2,1)

Pushups X2

Sit-upsX3

For Every Pull Up set do X2 pushups and X3 sit-ups

Example of Pyramid:

1 Pull Up Then 2 Push Ups then 3 Sit Ups
2 Pull Ups then 4 Push Ups and 6 Sit Ups
3 Pull Ups then 6 Push Ups then 9 Sit Ups

Cardio:
3 Mile Run at Medium Pace (8-10 Minute Miles) Goal
should be under 28 Minutes
Time: _______________

<u>Workout 26:</u>

3 Sets of 8-10 Reps Seated Overhead Dumbbell Press
Wt.____________________
3 Sets of 8-10 Reps Barbell Upright Rows
Wt.____________________
3 Sets of 8-10 Reps Seated Bent Over Rear Deltoid Raise
Wt.____________________
3 Sets of 8-10 Reps of Cable Face Pulls
Wt.____________________

2 Rounds for Time:
15 Large Arm Circles Forward
15 DB Front Raise
15 DB Side Raise
15 DB 45* Raise
15 Large Arm Circles Backwards
Time: ________________

Cardio:
Biking Pyramid 1-10-1
Stay at each level of resistance for 1 minute increasing to level 10 then decrease back to level 1 (Bike level 1 for 1 minute, then level 2 for one minute, then 3 for one minute- all the way to 10 and then back down to 1). Attempt to maintain above 100rpm at each level.
Distance: ________________

<u>Workout 27:</u>

3 Sets of 8-10 Reps Barbell Curl
Wt.______________
3 Sets of 8-10 Reps Skull Crushers
Wt.______________
3 Sets of 8-10 Reps of Close Grip Barbell Press
Wt.______________
3 Sets of 8-10 Reps of Dumbbell Bent Over Triceps Kickbacks
Wt.______________
3 Sets of 20 Diamond or Close Grip Push Ups
Wt.______________

2 Rounds for Time:
20 Dips (Assisted or Bench Dips for scale)
50 Crunches
20 Dumbbell Hammer Curls
50 Jumping Jacks
Time: ______________

Cardio:
20 Minutes of Stair Climber
10 Minutes on Bike at Medium Level (Maintain Over 100 RPM or Sub 5 Minute Mile)
Distance: ______________

<u>Workout 28:</u>

Cardio Day:
10X ¼ Mile Sprints in under 1:45 Per Sprint (60 Sec
Rest In between Sprints)
Completed Sprints: __ __ __ __ __ __ __ __ __ __
25 Burpees to Finish Cardio

<u>Workout 29:</u>

3 Sets of 8-10 Reps Barbell Bench Press
Wt._______________
3 Sets of 8-10 Reps Overhead Dumbbell Press
Wt._______________
3 Sets of 8-10 Reps Cable Triceps Extension
Wt._______________
3 Sets of 8-10 Reps Incline Bench Press
Wt._______________
3 Sets of 8-10 Reps Machine Chest Fly
Wt._______________
3 Sets of 8-10 Reps Standing Dumbbell Front Raise
Wt._______________

2 Rounds for Time:
10 Push Ups
20 Large Arm Circles Forward
20 Large Arm Circles Backward
10 Diamond Push Ups
20 Hanging Knee Raise
20 Russian Twists
Time: _______________

Cardio:
20 Min on Elliptical at HR 145-165
Distance: _______________

<u>Workout 30:</u>

3 Sets of 8-10 Reps Barbell Front Squats
Wt._______________
3 Sets of 8-10 (per leg) Dumbbell Lunges
Wt._______________
3 Sets of 8-10 Reps Machine Calf Raises
Wt._______________
3 Sets of 8-10 Reps Machine Leg Press
Wt._______________

2 Rounds for Time:
20 Box Jumps (Step Ups)
20 Machine Leg Extensions
20 Machine Leg Curls
20 Air Squats
Time: ______________

Cardio:
Biking Pyramid 1-10-1
Stay at each level of resistance for 1 minute increasing to level 10 then decrease back to level 1 (Bike level 1 for 1 minute, then level 2 for one minute, then 3 for one minute- all the way to 10 and then back down to 1). Attempt to maintain above 100rpm at each level.
Distance: ______________

<u>Workout 31</u>:

3 Sets of 8-10 Reps 1 and ¼ Bench Press
Wt.__________________
3 Sets of 8-10 Reps Machine Fly
Wt.__________________
3 Sets of 8-10 Reps Cable Fly (High to Low- position
cables at above shoulders)
Wt._______________
3 Sets of 8-10 Reps Cable Fly (Low to High- position
cables at ankles)
Wt._______________
3 Sets of 8-10 Reps Decline Bench Press
Wt.________________

2 Round for Time:
10 Diamond Push Ups
50 Crunches
20 Incline Push Ups
50 Russian Twists
30 Decline Push Ups
50 Flutter Kicks
Time: _______________

Cardio:
45 Minutes of Elliptical or Bike (HR 145-165)
Distance: _______________

<u>Workout 32:</u>

3 Sets of 8-10 Reps Dumbbell Hammer Curls
Wt.______________

3 Sets of 8-10 Reps Dumbbell Bent Over Triceps
Extension
Wt.______________

3 Sets of 8-10 Reps 1 and ¼ Straight Bar (Barbell) Bicep
Curls (¼ at the top portion of
movement)
Wt.______________

3 Sets of 8-10 Reps 1 ¼ Skull Crushers (¼ at the top
portion of movement)
Wt.______________

3 Sets of 8-10 Reps Single Cable Bicep Curls
Wt.______________

3 Sets of 8-10 Reps Single Cable Triceps Extension
Wt.______________

2 Rounds for Time:
20 Dips
20 KB Hammer Curls
20 Diamond Push Ups
50 Crunches
50 Flutter Kicks
Time: ______________

Cardio:
10 X 1:30 Minute Sprint on Level 10-12 (Sub 6-8
Minute Pace) 30 Seconds of Rest after each set
Completed Sprints: __ __ __ __ __ __ __ __ __ __

<u>Workout 33:</u>

3 Sets of 8-10 Reps Military Press
Wt.________________
3 Sets of 8-10 Reps DB Arnold Press
Wt.________________
3 Sets of 8-10 Reps DB Front Shoulder Raise
Wt.________________
3 Sets of 8-10 Reps DB Side Shoulder Raise
Wt.________________
3 Sets of 8-10 Reps DB Overhead Press
Wt.________________

2 Rounds for Time:
50 Small Arm Circles Forward
50 Small Arm Circles Backward
50 Crunches
50 Large Arm Circles Forward
50 Large Arm Circles Backward
50 Reverse Crunches
Time: ________________

Cardio:
2 Mile Run at 6:00-8:00 Minute per mile pace – Goal is
sub 12:00 minute completion
Time: ________________

Workout 34:

3 Sets of 8-10 Reps Weighted Pull Ups
Wt._______________
3 Sets of 8-10 Reps Cable Lat Push-downs
Wt._______________
3 Sets of 8-10 Reps Cable Seated Rows
Wt._______________
3 Sets of 8-10 Reps Machine Back Fly
Wt._______________
3 Sets of 8-10 Reps Bent Over Dumbbell Rows
Wt._______________

2 Rounds for Time:
10 Pull-ups
20 Push-ups
30 Core Twists
40 Bicycle Crunches
50 Crunches
Time: _______________

Cardio:
15 Minutes on Bike at RPM +100
Distance: _______________
15 Minutes on Elliptical at HR 145-165
Distance: _______________
15 Minutes on Stair climber

<u>Workout 35:</u>

3 Sets of 8-10 Reps Barbell Front Squats
Wt.________________
3 Sets of 8-10 Reps Per Single Leg Extension
Wt.________________
3 Sets of 8-10 Reps Per Single Leg Curl
Wt.________________
3 Sets of 8-10 Reps Weighted Seated Leg Press
Wt.________________
3 Sets of 8-10 Reps Machine Calf Raise
Wt.________________
3 Sets of 8-10 Reps Bench Split Squat Per Leg
Wt.________________

2 Rounds for Time:
10 Jumping Squats
10 Jumping Lunges
10 Bunny Hops (Toe Jumps)
50 Jumping Jacks
50 Flutter Kicks
Time: ________________

Cardio:
40 Minutes of Walking on Treadmill with Incline set at
12 or on highest setting
Distance: ____________

<u>Workout 36:</u>

3 Sets of 8-10 Reps Barbell Bicep Curls
Wt.___________________
20 Diamond Pushups
3 Sets of 8-10 Reps Barbell Laying Triceps Extension
Wt.___________________
20 Diamond Pushups
3 Sets of 8-10 Reps Seated Incline Dumbbell Curls
Wt.___________________
20 Diamond Pushups
3 Sets of 8-10 Reps Cable Overhead Triceps Extension
Wt.___________________
3 Sets of 8-10 Reps Seated Dumbbell Hammer Curls
Wt.___________________

2 Rounds for Time:
30 Second Plank
30 Bicycle Crunches
30 Second Left Oblique Plank
30 Crunches
30 Second Right Oblique Plank
30 Reverse Crunches
Time: _______________

Cardio:
1.5 Mile Run at 6:00-8:00 Minute Pace Per Mile
Time: _____________
Bike 15 Minutes at over 100 RPM (HR 145-165)
Distance: _____________
1.5 Mile Run at 6:00-8:00 Minute Pace Per Mile
Time: _____________

<u>Workout 37:</u>

3 Sets of 8-10 Reps Close Grip Barbell Bench Press
Wt.___________________
3 Sets of 8-10 Reps Incline Dumbbell Bench Press
Wt.___________________
3 Sets of 8-10 Reps Decline Dumbbell Bench Press
Wt.___________________
3 Sets of 8-10 Reps Cable Chest Fly
Wt.___________________
3 Sets of 8-10 Reps Weighted Dips
Wt.___________________

2 Rounds for Time:
10 Burpees or Up/Downs
20 Pushups
30 Core Twists (Russian Twists)
Time: _______________

Cardio:
45 Min on Elliptical maintaining HR between 145-165
Distance: _______________

<u>Workout 38:</u>

3 Sets of 8-10 Reps Dumbbell Split Squats (8-10 per leg)
Wt._______________
3 Sets of 8-10 Reps 1 Leg Kettle Bell Deadlift (8-10 per leg)
Wt._______________
3 Sets of 8-10 Reps Leg Extension (Hold at top 2 sec)
Wt._______________
3 Sets of 8-10 Reps Leg Curls (Hold at top 2 sec)
Wt._______________
3 Sets of 8-10 Reps Machine Leg Press (4 Count Down)
Wt._______________
3 Sets of 8-10 Reps Machine Calf Raise (Hold at top 2 sec)
Wt._______________

3 Rounds for Time:
20 Dumbbell Step Ups
20 Dumbbell Calf Raise
20 Mountain Climbers
20 Reverse Crunches
20 Jumping Jacks
Time: _______________

Cardio:
10 X 2:00 Sprint on Level 8-10 or 6:00-8:00 Min. Mile Pace (Incline Level 8-10)
Sets: __ __ __ __ __ __ __ __ __ __
20 Minutes Elliptical (HR 145-165)
Distance: _______________

<u>Workout 39:</u>

3 Sets of 8-10 Reps Lat Pull Down Close Grip
Wt.______________
3 Sets of 8-10 Reps Seated Military Press
Wt.______________
3 Sets of 8-10 Reps Seated Cable Row
Wt.______________
3 Sets of 8-10 Reps Machine Shoulder Press
Wt.______________
3 Sets of 8-10 Reps Barbell Shrugs
Wt.______________
3 Sets of 8-10 Reps Machine Back Fly
Wt.______________

3 Rounds for Time:
10 Pull-Ups
20 Standing Knees-to-elbow cross
10 Dumbbell Overhead Press
20 Flutter Kicks
10 Pushups
20 Bicycle Crunches
Time: ____________

Cardio:
3 Mile Jog at 8:00-10:00 Min Mile Pace Per Mile (Goal
Completion Time: 24 Minutes)
Time: ____________
1 Mile Cool Down Walk at Incline Level 10 on
Treadmill

<u>Workout 40:</u>

3 Sets of 8-10 Reps Barbell Preacher Curls (Machine if needed)
Wt.______________
3 Sets of 8-10 Reps Bench Press (3 Count Down)
Wt.______________
3 Sets of 8-10 Reps Barbell Skull Crushers
Wt.______________
3 Sets of 8-10 Reps Machine Chest Fly
Wt.______________
3 Sets of 8-10 Reps Dumbbell Hammer Curls
Wt.______________
3 Sets of 8-10 Reps Dumbbell Triceps Extension
Wt.______________

3 Rounds for Time:
15 Kettle Bell Hammer Curls
15 Kettle Bell Overhead Triceps Extension
15 Kettle Bell Swings
15 Kettle Bell High Pulls
30 Flutter Kicks
30 Bicycle Crunches
Time: ___________

Cardio:
20 Minutes Stair Climber
20 Minutes Elliptical (HR 145-165)
Distance: _________
20 Minutes Bike RPM +100 Distance: ___________

<u>Workout 41:</u>

3 Sets of 8-10 Reps 1 Leg Machine Extensions (8-10 per leg)
Wt.____________
3 Sets of 8-10 Reps 1 Leg Machine Curls (8-10 per leg)
Wt.____________
3 Sets of 8-10 Reps Barbell Shrugs (2 Second hold at top) Wt.____________
3 Sets of 8-10 Reps 1 and ¼ Barbell Squats
Wt.____________
3 Sets of 8-10 Reps Barbell Hang Clean
Wt.____________
3 Sets of 8-10 Reps Machine Calf Raise
Wt.____________

3 Rounds for Time:
30 Air Squats
30 Second Kettle Bell Farmers Carry
30 Walking Lunges
30 Second Front Plank
30 Second Side Plank (Each Side)
Time: ____________

Cardio:
20 Minutes Stair Climber
20 Minutes Bike RPM +100
Distance: ____________
20 Minutes Walking at Incline 10-12 on Treadmill
Distance: ____________

Workout 42:

3 Sets of 8-10 Reps Dumbbell Arnold Press
Wt._________________
3 Sets of 8-10 Reps Seated Lateral Dumbbell Raise
Wt._________________
3 Sets of 8-10 Reps Bent Over Dumbbell Row
Wt._________________
3 Sets of 8-10 Reps Machine Lat Pull Down
Wt._________________
3 Sets of 8-10 Reps Cable Face Pulls
Wt._________________
3 Sets of 8-10 Reps Cable Back Fly
Wt._________________

3 Rounds for Time:
10 Pull Ups
20 Push Ups
30 V-Ups
Time: _____________

Cardio:
2000 Meter Rowing Machine Row (Goal= Under 20 Minutes)
Time: _____________
10 X ¼ Mile Sprints (Goal= Under 2 Minutes Per ¼ Mile) 45 Second Rest in between sets
Completed Sets: __ __ __ __ __ __ __ __ __ __

<u>Workout 43</u>:

3 Sets of 8-10 Reps Reverse Grip Barbell Bench Press
Wt.________________
3 Sets of 8-10 Reps Close Grip Barbell Bench Press
Wt.________________
3 Sets of 8-10 Reps Seated Dumbbell Curls
Wt.________________
3 Sets of 8-10 Reps Seated Dumbbell Overhead Triceps
Extension Wt.________________
3 Sets of 8-10 Reps Cable Fly
Wt.________________
3 Sets of 8-10 Reps Decline Barbell Bench Press
Wt.________________

3 Rounds for Time:
30 Push Ups
30 Russian Twists (Core Twists)
30 Jumping Jacks
30 Flutter Kicks
30 Mountain Climbers
Time: ____________

Cardio:
25 Box Jumps
Time: ____________
25 Burpees
Time: ____________
2 Mile Jog at 8:00-10:00 Minute per Mile Pace
Time: ____________
2 Mile Bike Ride at 100+ RPM Time: ____________

<u>Workout 44:</u>

3 Sets of 8-10 Reps Machine Leg Extension (2 Sec Hold at Top)
Wt.________________
3 Sets of 8-10 Reps Machine Leg Curls (2 Sec Hold at Top)
Wt.________________
3 Sets of 8-10 Reps Machine Leg Press
Wt.________________
3 Sets of 8-10 Reps Barbell Front Squats
Wt.________________
3 Sets of 8-10 Reps Barbell Calf Raise
Wt.________________
3 Sets of 8-10 Reps Machine Calf Raise
Wt.________________

3 Rounds for Time:
20 Dumbbell Box Step Ups
20 Dumbbell Lunges (10 Per Leg)
20 Dumbbell Thrusters
20 V-Ups
Time: ___________

Cardio:
5 Mile Run on Incline 8 on Treadmill (Goal= Under 45 Minutes or Sub 8:00 Minute Mile Pace Per Mile)
Time: ___________

<u>Workout 45:</u>

3 Sets of 8-10 Reps Standing Barbell Curls
Wt._________________
3 Sets of 8-10 Reps Skull Crushers
Wt._________________
3 Sets of 8-10 Reps Cable Bicep Curls
Wt._________________
3 Sets of 8-10 Reps Cable Triceps Extensions
Wt._________________
3 Sets of 8-10 Reps Dumbbell Hammer Curls
Wt._________________
3 Sets of 8-10 Reps Bent Over Dumbbell Triceps
Extension
Wt._________________

3 Rounds for Time:
20 Dips
20 Flutter Kicks
20 Close Grip Push Ups (Diamond)
20 Hanging Knee Raise
Time: ___________

Cardio:
10 X ¼ Mile Sprints (Goal= Under 2 Minutes Per ¼
Mile 45 Second Rest in between sets)
Completed Sets: __ __ __ __ __ __ __ __ __ __
1 Mile Sprint (Goal=6:00 Minute Mile)
Time: ___________

<u>Workout 46:</u>

3 Sets of 8-10 Reps Dumbbell Standing Front Raise
Wt.________________
3 Sets of 8-10 Reps Dumbbell Standing Lateral Raise
Wt.________________
3 Sets of 8-10 Reps Seated Dumbbell Overhead Press
Wt.________________
3 Sets of 8-10 Reps Barbell Shrugs
Wt.________________
3 Sets of 8-10 Reps Barbell High Pull
Wt.________________
3 Sets of 8-10 Reps Cable Face Pulls
Wt.________________

3 Rounds for Time:
30 Large Arm Circles Forward
30 Large Arm Circles Backward
30 Russian Twists (Core Twists)
30 Overhead Air Press
30 Second Plank
Time: ___________

Cardio:
45 Minutes on Elliptical (145-165 HR)
Distance: ___________

<u>Workout 47:</u>

3 Sets of 8-10 Reps Lat Pull Downs
Wt._________________
3 Sets of 8-10 Reps Bent Over Dumbbell Rows
Wt._________________
3 Sets of 8-10 Reps Seated Machine Rows
Wt._________________
3 Sets of 8-10 Reps Machine Back Fly
Wt._________________
3 Sets of 8-10 Reps Bent Over Barbell Rows
Wt._________________
3 Sets of 8-10 Reps Barbell Deadlifts
Wt._________________

3 Rounds for Time:
10 Pull Ups
500-meter Rowing Machine Row
20 Reverse Flutter Kicks
20 Push Ups
Time: ___________

Cardio:
6 X ¼ Mile Sprint (Goal= Under 2:00 Minutes per Sprint)
Sets: __ __ __ __ __ __
4 X ½ Mile Sprint (Goal= Under 3:30 Minutes Per Sprint)
Sets: __ __ __ __
10 Minutes on Bicycle RPM 100+
Distance: _________

<u>Workout 48:</u>

3 Sets of 8-10 Reps Incline Bench Press
Wt.________________
3 Sets of 8-10 Reps Cable Chest Fly or Machine Fly
Wt.________________
3 Sets of 8-10 Reps Decline Dumbbell Bench Press
Wt.________________
3 Sets of 8-10 Reps Dumbbell Hammer Curls
Wt.________________
3 Sets of 8-10 Reps Dumbbell Triceps Extension
Wt.________________
3 Sets of 8-10 Reps Cable Bicep Curls
Wt.________________

3 Rounds for Time (Abs):
20 Russian Core Twists
20 Bicycle Crunches
20 Laying Leg Lifts
20 Ball Crunches
Time: ___________

3 Rounds for Time:
10 Lightweight Bench Press
30 Second Ab Plank
Time: ___________
Cardio:
10 Sets of 30 Seconds of Running / 30 Seconds Rest
(Pace 8-10 or 6-8 min Mile)
Sets: __ __ __ __ __ __ __ __ __ __
15 Minutes Stair Climber
500 Meter Row on Rowing Machine Time: ___________

<u>Workout 49:</u>

3 Sets of 8-10 Seated Leg Ext. (Machine)
Wt._______________
3 Sets of 8-10 Seated Machine Calf Raises
Wt._______________
3 Sets of 8-10 Seated Leg Curl (Machine)
Wt._______________
3 Sets of 8-10 Seated Leg Press
Wt._______________
3 Sets of 8-10 Barbell Squats
Wt._______________
3 Sets of 8-10 Romanian Barbell Deadlift
Wt._______________

3 Rounds for Time:
20 Walking Lunges (10 Each Leg)
20 V-Ups
10 Jumping Air Squats
30 Russian Twists
30 Flutter Kicks
30 Jumping Jacks
Time: __________

Cardio:
20 Min. on Elliptical maintaining HR between 145-165
Distance: _______________
20 Min. on Treadmill walking at Level 10-12 Incline
Distance: _______________

<u>Workout 50:</u>

3 Sets of 8-10 Reps Cable Face Pull
Wt._______________
3 Sets of 8-10 Reps Cable Lat Pull Downs
Wt._______________
3 Sets of 8-10 Reps of Weighted Pull Ups
Wt._______________
3 Sets of 8-10 Reps Machine Back Fly
Wt._______________
3 Sets of 8-10 Seated Cable Machine Rows
Wt._______________

3 Rounds for Time:
20 Bent over Dumbbell rows (10 Each Arm)
20 Incline Pushups
20 Dumbbell Shrugs
20 Russian Twists / Core Twist
20 Flutter Kicks
Time: ___________

Cardio:
1000 meters on the Rowing Machine
Time: ___________
20 minutes on Stair Climbers
10 Minutes on Bike RPM +100
Distance: ___________

<u>Workout 51:</u>

3 Sets of 8-10 Reps Seated Overhead Dumbbell Press
Wt.__________________
3 Sets of 8-10 Reps Barbell Upright Rows
Wt.__________________
3 Sets of 8-10 Reps Seated Bent Over Rear Deltoid
Raise
Wt.__________________
3 Sets of 8-10 Reps Barbell Shrug
Wt.__________________

3 Rounds for Time:
15 DB Front Raise
15 DB Side Raise
15 DB 45* Raise
15 Kettle Bell Swings
15 Kettle Bell Overhead Press
Time: ___________

Cardio:
Biking Pyramid 1-10-1
Stay at each level of resistance for 1 minute increasing to
level 10 then decrease back to level 1 (Bike level 1 for 1
minute, then level 2 for one minute, then 3 for one
minute- all the way to 10 and then back down to 1)
Maintain 100rpm at each level. Distance: ___________

1 Mile Sprint on Treadmill (Goal 6:00-7:00 minute pace)
Time: ___________

<u>Workout 52:</u>

3 Sets of 8-10 Reps Cable Bicep Curls
Wt._______________
3 Sets of 8-10 Reps Cable Triceps Extensions
Wt._______________
3 Sets of 8-10 Reps Machine Preacher Curls
Wt._______________
3 Sets of 8-10 Reps Machine Triceps Extension
Wt._______________
3 Sets of 8-10 Reps Barbell Bicep Curls
Wt._______________

3 Rounds for Time:
10 Dumbbell Hammer Curls (10 each arm)
10 Bench Dips
10 Dumbbell Curls (10 each arm)
10 Barbell Skull Crushers
Time: ___________

2 Rounds for Time:
20 Ball Crunches
20 Hanging Knee Raises
20 Russian Twists
20 Flutter Kicks
Time: ___________

Cardio:
30 Minute Treadmill Cool Down Walk on Incline Level
10-12
Distance: _____________

<u>Workout 53:</u>

Max Repetitions (1 Minute Break Between Workouts)

2 Minutes of Mountain Climbers
Reps: ___________
2 Minutes of Ball Crunches
Reps: ___________
2 Minutes of Jumping Lunges
Reps: ___________
2 Minutes of Jumping Jacks
Reps: ___________
2 Minutes of Side-to-Side Hops
Reps: ___________
2 Minutes of Air Squats
Reps: ___________
2 Minutes of Knee Push-Ups
Reps: ___________

Cardio:
3-Mile Slow Jog (Incline Level 5-6 with 10-11:00
Minute Mile Pace) Goal Time= 30 Minutes
Time: ___________

Workout 54:

3 Sets of 8-10 Reps Barbell Bench Press
Wt.__________________
3 Sets of 8-10 Reps Seated Military Overhead Press
Wt.__________________
3 Sets of 8-10 Reps Cable Triceps Extension
Wt.__________________
3 Sets of 8-10 Reps Dumbbell Bicep Curls
Wt.__________________
3 Sets of 8-10 Reps Cable Bicep Curls (Single Arm at a
Time)
Wt.__________________

3 Rounds for Time:
10 Dips
10 Dumbbell Front Raise
10 Overhead Dumbbell Triceps Extension
20 V-Ups
20 Flutter Kicks
20 DB Hammer Curls (10 Each Arm)
Time: ____________

Cardio:
Run-
2 X ½ mile at 4:00min each ½ mile. Target Pace set as 8-
minute mile on Treadmill (60 Sec Rest Between each ½
Mile) Sets Completed: __ __
4 X ¼ Mile at 2:00min each ¼ mile. Target Pace set as
8-minute mile pace on Treadmill (60 Sec Rest Between
each 1/4 mile) Sets Completed: __ __ __ __

<u>Workout 55:</u>

3 Sets of 8-10 Reps Machine Leg Extensions
Wt.______________
3 Sets of 8-10 Reps Machine Leg Curls
Wt.______________
3 Sets of 8-10 Reps Machine Calf Raises
Wt.______________
3 Sets of 8-10 Reps Machine Leg Press
Wt.______________
3 Sets of 8-10 Reps Cable Face Pulls
Wt.______________
3 Sets of 8-10 Reps Barbell Shrugs (2 Sec Hold at Top)
Wt.______________

3 Rounds for Time:
20 1 and ¼ air squats
20 Jumping Lunges
20 Air Calf Raises
30 Jumping Jacks
Time: __________

Cardio:
20 Minutes of Stair Climbers (Stair Master)
20 Minutes of Elliptical
Distance: __________
20 Minutes of Rowing on the Rowing Machine
Distance: __________

<u>Workout 56:</u>

3 Sets of 8-10 Reps Cable Lat Pull Down
Wt.________________
3 Sets of 8-10 Reps Machine Bicep Curls
Wt.________________
3 Sets of 8-10 Reps Machine Triceps Extension
Wt.________________
3 Sets of 8-10 Pull Ups
Wt.________________
3 Sets of 8-10 Reps Bent Over Dumbbell Rows
Wt.________________
3 Sets of 8-10 Reps Seated Overhead Dumbbell Press
(Arnold Press if able)
Wt.________________

3 Rounds for Time:
15 Cable Tri Extensions
15 Cable Bicep Cable Curls
15 Dips
15 Push Ups
15 Burpees
Time: ___________

Cardio:
1.5 Mile Sprint at Level 8-10 (Between 6:00-8:00 minute
mile pace)
Time: ___________
20 Minutes on Stationary Bike RPM +100
Distance: ___________

<u>Workout 57:</u>

Cardio Day
Biking Pyramid 1-10-1
Stay at each level of resistance for 1 minute increasing to
level 10 then decrease back to level 1 (Bike level 1 for 1
minute, then level 2 for one minute, then 3 for one
minute- all the way to 10 and then back down to 1).
Attempt to maintain 100rpm at each level.
Distance: ___________

10 Sets of 30 Seconds of Running / 30 Seconds Rest
(Incline level 12, Speed Level 8-10 or 6-8 min Mile
Pace)
Sets Completed: __ __ __ __ __ __ __ __ __ __
15 Minutes of Stair Climber
500 Meter Sprint Row on Rowing Machine
Time: ___________

<u>Workout 58:</u>

3 Sets of 8-10 Reps Barbell Close Grip Bench Press
Wt.________________
3 Sets of 8-10 Reps Incline Dumbbell Bench Press
Wt.________________
3 Sets of 8-10 Reps Decline Dumbbell Bench Press
Wt.________________
3 Sets of 8-10 Reps Dips
Wt.________________
3 Sets of 8-10 Reps Hammer Dumbbell Curls
Wt.________________
3 Sets of 8-10 Reps Bent Over Dumbbell Triceps
Extension
Wt.________________

3 Rounds for Time:
10 Standing Cable Fly Angled Down
10 Standing Cable Fly Angled Up
10 Standing Cable Fly
10 Cable Triceps Extension
10 Cable Bicep Curl
Time: ___________

Cardio:
20 Min of Elliptical Machine HR 145-165 or at sub 6
min pace
Distance: ___________
20 Minutes on Stair Climber

<u>Workout 59:</u>

3 Sets of 8-10 Reps Barbell Squats
Wt._________________
3 Sets of 8-10 Reps (Per Leg) Walking Dumbbell
Lunges
Wt._________________
3 Sets of 8-10 Reps of Barbell Romanian Deadlift
Wt._______________
3 Sets of 8-10 Reps Machine Calf Raise
Wt._______________

3 Rounds for Time:
10 Burpees
20 Russian Twists
20 Hanging Knee Raise
20 Crunches
30 Sec Plank Left Side
30 Sec Plank Right Side
50 Jumping Jacks
Time: ___________

Cardio:
15 Minutes of Bike (Medium Level/ Maintain RPM at
100)
Distance: ______________
15 Minute Run (Goal is 1.5-2.0 Miles) Incline Level 10
Distance: ______________

<u>Workout 60:</u>

3 Sets of 8-10 Reps Pull Ups
Wt._________________
3 Sets of 8-10 Reps Barbell Bent over Rows
Wt._________________
3 Sets of 8-10 Reps Cable Face Pull
Wt._________________
3 Sets of 8-10 Reps Machine Back Fly
Wt._________________
3 Sets of 8-10 Reps Barbell High Pull
Wt._________________

3 Rounds for Time:
20 Seated Dumbbell Overhead Press
20 Dumbbell Shrugs
20 Dumbbell Front Raise
20 Dumbbell Shrugs
20 Push Ups
Time: ___________

Cardio:
30 Minutes on the Elliptical or Cardio of Choice
Distance: ____________

<u>Workout 61:</u>

3 Sets of 8-10 Reps Dumbbell Bench Press
Wt.________________
3 Sets of 8-10 Reps Cable Triceps Extension
Wt.________________
3 Sets of 8-10 Reps Laying Dumbbell Chest Fly
Wt.________________
3 Sets of 8-10 Reps Seated Dumbbell Hammer Curl
Wt.________________
3 Sets of 8-10 Reps Seated Overhead Dumbbell
Triceps Extension Wt.________________
3 Sets of 8-10 Reps Decline Barbell Bench Press
Wt.________________

3 Rounds for Time:
10 Barbell Curls
20 Push Ups
10 Barbell Skull Crushers
20 Push Ups
10 Barbell Reverse Curls
20 Crunches
Time: __________

Biking Pyramid 1-10-1
Stay at each level of resistance for 1 minute increasing to
level 10 then decrease back to level 1 (Bike level 1 for 1
minute, then level 2 for one minute, then 3 for one
minute- all the way to level 10 and then go back down to
1). Attempt to maintain 100rpm at each increasing level.
Distance: ____________
20 Minutes Elliptical Distance: ____________

Workout 62:

3 Sets of 8-10 Reps Leg Extensions
Wt.________________
3 Sets of 8-10 Reps Leg Curls
Wt.________________
3 Sets of 8-10 Reps Machine Leg Press
Wt.________________
3 Sets of 8-10 Reps Barbell Shrugs
Wt.________________
3 Sets of 8-10 Reps Machine Calf Raise
Wt.________________
3 Sets of 8-10 Reps Dumbbell Split Squats
Wt.________________

3 Rounds for Time:
20 1 and ¼ Air Squats
20 Crunches
20 Bodyweight Lunges (10 Each Leg)
20 Russian Twists
20 Jumping Jacks
20 V-Ups
Time: ____________

Cardio:
2 X 1 Mile Sprints (Level 8-10 or 6:00-8:00 Min Mile
Pace) – 1 Minute rest between miles
Sets Completed: __ __
1000 Meter Row on the Rowing Machine
Time: ____________
20 Burpees

<u>Workout 63:</u>

3 Sets of 8-10 Reps Seated Cable Rows
Wt.______________
3 Sets of 8-10 Reps Cable Face Pulls
Wt.______________
3 Sets of 8-10 Reps Cable Lat Push Down
Wt.______________
3 Sets of 8-10 Reps Seated Dumbbell Overhead Press
Wt.______________
3 Sets of 8-10 Reps Bent Over Dumbbell Rows
Wt.______________

3 Rounds for Time:
10 Pull Ups
10 Dumbbell Side Raise
30 Hanging Knee Raise
30 Russian Twists
10 Dumbbell 45* Raise
10 Dumbbell Front Raise
Time: ___________

Cardio:
2 X ½ Mile Sprints (Goal Pace 3:00 minutes per ½ mile)
60 Second Rest Between ½ Miles
Sets Completed: __ __
20 Minutes of Speed Walking on Treadmill at #12 Incline
Distance: ______________

<u>Workout 64:</u>

3 Sets of 8-10 Reps Barbell Decline Bench Press
Wt.__________________
3 Sets of 8-10 Reps Barbell Bicep Curls
Wt.__________________
3 Sets of 8-10 Reps Machine Chest Fly
Wt.__________________
3 Sets of 8-10 Reps Cable Triceps Extension
Wt.__________________
3 Sets of 8-10 Reps Barbell Incline Bench Press
Wt.__________________
3 Sets of 8-10 Reps Dumbbell Laying Close Grip Bench Press
Wt.__________________
3 Sets of 8-10 Reps Dumbbell Bicep Curls
Wt.__________________

3 Rounds for Time:
20 Incline Push Ups
20 Russian Twists
20 Bench Dips
20 Crunches
20 Bicycle Crunches
Time: __________

Cardio:
10 Sets of 30 Seconds Running / 15 Seconds Rest
(Incline level 12, Pace 8-10 or 6-8 min Mile pace)
Sets Completed: __ __ __ __ __ __ __ __ __ __
20 Minutes Walking on Incline Level 12 on Treadmill
Distance: ______________

<u>Workout 65:</u>

3 Sets of 8-10 Reps Barbell Front Squats
Wt.___________________
3 Sets of 8-10 Reps Barbell Shrugs
Wt.___________________
3 Sets of 8-10 Reps Leg Ext (2 Sec Hold at Top)
Wt.___________________
3 Sets of 8-10 Reps Leg Curl (2 Sec Hold at Top)
Wt.___________________
3 Sets of 8-10 Reps Hang Clean
Wt.___________________
3 Sets of 8-10 Reps Machine Leg Press
Wt.___________________
3 Sets of 8-10 Reps Machine Calf Raise
Wt.___________________

3 Rounds for Time:
20 Air Squats
20 Box Jumps
20 Walking Lunges (10 Each Leg)
20 Laying Leg Lifts
20 Bunny Hops
20 V-Ups
Time: ____________

Cardio:
20 Minutes of Running at Level 6 or 10 Min Per Mile
Pace but set on Incline 12
Distance: ______________
20 Minutes of Stair Climber
10 Minutes of Bike 100+ RPM Distance: ______________

<u>Workout 66:</u>

3 Sets of 8-10 Reps Dumbbell Bent over Rows (per arm)
Wt.______________
3 Sets of 8-10 Reps Barbell Military Overhead Press
Wt.______________
3 Sets of 8-10 Reps Cable Lat Pull Down
Wt.______________
3 Sets of 8-10 Reps Standing Cable Front Raise
Wt.______________
3 Sets of 8-10 Reps Machine/Cable Back Fly
Wt.______________
3 Sets of 8-10 Reps Pull Ups
Wt.______________

3 Rounds for Time:
20 Small Arm Circles Forward
20 Overhead Air Press
20 Small Arm Circles Backward
20 Overhead Air Press
20 Large Arm Circles Forward
20 Large Arm Circles Backward
20 Russian Twists
Time: __________

Cardio:
2 X ¼ Mile at 1:30min pace (30 Sec Rest Between 1/4
miles) Sets Completed: __ __
4 X 1/8mile at :45 seconds pace (30 Sec Rest Between
Rounds) Sets Completed: __ __
10 Minute Cool Down Walk on Incline 12
Distance: ______________

<u>Workout 67:</u>

3 Sets of 8-10 Reps Close Grip Barbell Bench Press
Wt.________________
3 Sets of 8-10 Reps Dumbbell Hammer Curls
Wt.________________
3 Sets of 8-10 Reps Overhead Dumbbell Tri Extension
Wt.________________
3 Sets of 8-10 Reps Barbell Reverse Bicep Curl
Wt.________________
3 Sets of 8-10 Reps Weighted Dips
Wt.________________
3 Sets of 8-10 Reps Incline Dumbbell Bench Press
Wt.________________
3 Sets of 8-10 Reps (Each Arm) Single Arm Cable
Triceps Extension
Wt.________________
3 Sets of 8-10 Reps (Each Arm) Single Arm Cable Bicep
Curl Wt.________________

3 Rounds for Time:
20 Burpees
20 Flutter Kicks
20 Laying Superman
20 Crunches
20 Good Mornings (Standing Hip Hinge)
20 Push Ups
Time: ___________

Cardio:
20 Minutes of Stair Climber at Medium Speed
1500-Meter Row Time: ___________

$$\underline{\text{Workout 68:}}$$

3 Sets of 8-10 Reps Barbell Front Squats
Wt._______________
3 Sets of 8-10 Reps Barbell Shrugs
Wt._______________
3 Sets of 8-10 Reps Leg Extension
Wt._______________
3 Sets of 8-10 Reps Leg Curls
Wt._______________
3 Sets of 8-10 Reps Calf Raises
Wt._______________
3 Sets of 8-10 Reps Machine Leg Press
Wt._______________
3 Sets of 8-10 Reps Cable Shrugs
Wt._______________

3 Rounds for Time:
20 Box Jumps
20 Flutter Kicks
20 Walking Dumbbell Lunges
20 Jumping Jacks
20 V-Ups
Time: ___________

Cardio:
20-Minute Elliptical at HR 145-165 (Sub 6 Minute Pace)
Distance: _______________
20-Minute Moderate Jog on Incline Level 8 (9:00-10:00 minute per mile goal pace)
Distance: _______________

<u>Workout 69</u>:

Cardio Day:
1 Mile Run at Slow Pace (10:00-11:00 Minute Pace)
Time: ___________
1000 Meters on Rowing Machine
Time: ___________
50 V-Ups
1 Mile Run at Moderate Pace (8:00-10:00 Minute Pace)
Time: ___________
50 Sit Ups
1000 Meters on Rowing Machine
Time: ___________
1 Mile Run at Fast Pace (6:00-8:00 Minute Pace)
Time: ___________
50 Russian Twists
1000 Meters on Rowing Machine
Time: ___________

Workout 70:

3 Sets of 8-10 Reps 1 and ¼ Barbell Bench Press
Wt._______________
3 Sets of 8-10 Reps Machine Chest Fly
Wt._______________
3 Sets of 8-10 Reps Dips
Wt._______________
3 Sets of 8-10 Reps Barbell Incline Bench Press
Wt._______________
3 Sets of 8-10 Reps Dumbbell Bicep Curls
Wt._______________
3 Sets of 8-10 Reps Dumbbell Decline Bench Press (2
Sec Hold at Top) Wt._______________
3 Sets of 8-10 Reps Machine Bicep Curls
Wt._______________
3 Sets of 8-10 Reps Machine Triceps Extension
Wt._______________

3 Rounds for Time:
20 Push Ups
20 Decline Sit Ups
20 Med Ball Twists
20 Med Ball Curls
20 DB Overhead Triceps Extension
20 Flutter Kicks
Time: ___________

Cardio:
5-Mile Bike Ride at Sub 6 Minute Pace Per Mile (Goal
Time is 30:00 minutes or Less) Time: ___________

<u>Workout 71:</u>

3 Rounds for Time:
20 Jumping Air Squats
20 Russian Twists
20 Jumping Lunges
20 Laying Leg Lifts
20 Dirty Dogs (Per Leg)
20 Donkey Kicks (Per Leg)
Time: ___________

3 Sets of 8-10 Reps Machine Leg Extensions (2 Sec Hold at Top and 4 Count Back Down)
Wt._______________
3 Sets of 8-10 Reps Machine Leg Curls (2 Sec Hold at Top and 4 Count Back Down)
Wt._______________
3 Sets of 8-10 Reps Machine Calf Raise (2 Sec Hold at Top) Wt._______________
3 Sets of 8-10 Reps Machine Leg Press
Wt._______________
3 Sets of 8-10 Reps Barbell 1 ¼ Squats
Wt._______________
3 Sets of 8-10 Reps of Barbell Calf Raise
Wt._______________

Cardio:
2000-Meter Row on Rowing Machine
Time: ___________
100 Jumping Jacks
1 Mile Run at 6:00-8:00 Mile/Minute Pace
Time: ___________

<u>Workout 72:</u>

Pull/Push/Sit-up Pyramid
1-10-1 of Pull Ups (1,2,3,4,5,6,7,8,9,10,9,8,7,6,5,4,3,2,1)
Pushups X2
Sit-ups X3
For Every Pull Up set do x2 pushups and x3 sit-ups
Time: ___________

Cardio:
3 Mile Run at Medium Pace (8-10 Minute per Mile pace)
Goal should be under 28 Minutes Incline Level 7
Time: ___________

<u>Workout 73:</u>

3 Sets of 8-10 Reps Seated Overhead Dumbbell Press
Wt._________________
3 Sets of 8-10 Reps KB Swings
Wt._________________
3 Sets of 8-10 Reps Barbell Upright Rows
Wt._______________
3 Sets of 8-10 Reps Seated Bent Over Rear Deltoid
Raise Wt._________________
3 Sets of 8-10 Reps of Cable Face Pulls
Wt._________________
3 Sets of 1 Minute DB Farmers Carry Walk
Wt._________________

3 Rounds for Time:
15 Large Arm Circles Forward
15 DB Front Raise
15 DB Side Raise
15 DB 45* Raise
15 Large Arm Circles Backwards
30 V-Ups
30 Russian Twists
Time: ___________

Cardio:
Biking Pyramid 1-10-1
Stay at each level of resistance for 1 minute increasing to
level 10 then decrease back to level 1. Attempt to
maintain 100 rpm at each level.
Distance: ____________
1 Mile Jog at 8-10 Minute Pace Time: ___________

<u>Workout 74:</u>

3 Sets of 8-10 Reps Barbell Curl
Wt._______________
3 Sets of 8-10 Reps Skull Crushers
Wt._______________
3 Sets of 8-10 Reps of Close Grip Barbell Bench Press
Wt._______________
3 Sets of 8-10 Reps of Dumbbell Triceps Bent over
Kickbacks Wt._______________
3 Sets of 20 Diamond or Close Grip Push Ups
3 Sets of 8-10 Reps Cable Bicep Curls
Wt._______________
3 Sets of 8-10 Reps Cable Triceps Extension
Wt._______________

3 Rounds for Time:
20 Dips (Assisted or Bench Dips for scale)
50 Crunches
20 Dumbbell Hammer Curls
50 Jumping Jacks
20 Burpees
Time: ___________

Cardio:
20 Minutes of Stair Climber
10 Minutes on Bike at Medium Level (Over 100 RPM)
Distance: ___________
10 X 1 minute Sprints (5-6 Minute/Mile Pace on
Treadmill) at Level 12 Incline
Sets Completed: __ __ __ __ __ __ __ __ __ __

Workout 75:

Cardio Day:
2000 Meter Rowing Machine
Time: ___________
10 X ¼ Mile Sprints goal under 1:45 Per Sprint (60 Sec Rest In between Sprints)
Sets Completed: __ __ __ __ __ __ __ __ __ __
25 Burpees
10 Minute Walk at Level 12 Incline for Cool Down
Distance: ___________

<u>Workout 76:</u>

3 Sets of 8-10 Reps Barbell Bent Over Rows
Wt._______________
3 Sets of 8-10 Reps Overhead Dumbbell Press
Wt._______________
3 Sets of 8-10 Reps Cable Face Pulls
Wt._______________
3 Sets of 8-10 Reps Cable Lat Push Down
Wt._______________
3 Sets of 8-10 Reps Machine Shoulder Raise
Wt._______________
3 Sets of 8-10 Reps Standing Dumbbell Front Raise
Wt._______________

3 Rounds for Time:
10 Push Ups
20 Large Arm Circles Forward
20 Large Arm Circles Backward
10 Hand-Stand Push Ups (Scaled if needed)
20 Hanging Knee Raise
20 Russian Twists
Time: _______________

Cardio:
20 Min on Elliptical at HR 145-165
Distance: _______________
10 X 1 Minute Sprints on Level 12 Incline (5:00-6:00
Minute Mile Pace)
Sets Completed: __ __ __ __ __ __ __ __ __ __

<u>Workout 77:</u>

3 Sets of 8-10 Reps Barbell 1 ¼ Front Squats
Wt.________________
3 Sets of 8-10 (per leg) Dumbbell Lunges
Wt.________________
3 Sets of 8-10 Reps Machine Calf Raises
Wt.________________
3 Sets of 8-10 Reps Machine Leg Press
Wt.________________
3 Sets of 8-10 Reps Romanian Deadlifts
Wt.________________

3 Rounds for Time:
20 Band Donkey Kicks (Cable Machine if No bands)
20 Band Dirty Dogs (Cable if No bands)
20 Box Jumps (Step Ups for Scale)
20 Machine Leg Extensions
20 Machine Leg Curls
20 Air Squats
Time: __________

Cardio:
5 Mile Walk Incline Level 12 on Treadmill
Time: __________

<u>Workout 78:</u>

3 Sets of 8-10 Reps 1 and ¼ Bench Press
Wt._________________
3 Sets of 8-10 Reps Cable Fly
Wt._________________
3 Sets of 8-10 Reps Cable Decline Press (High to Low-
position cables at above shoulders)
Wt._________________
3 Sets of 8-10 Reps Cable Incline Press (Low to High-
position cables at ankles)
Wt._________________
3 Sets of 8-10 Reps Decline Bench Press
Wt._________________

3 Rounds for Time:
50 Jumping Jacks
30 Diamond Push Ups
50 Crunches
30 Incline Push Ups
50 Russian Twists
30 Decline Push Ups
50 Flutter Kicks
Time: ___________

Cardio:
Row 1000 Meters to get HR elevated
Time: ___________
45 Minutes of Elliptical Machine (HR 145-165)
Distance: ___________

<u>Workout 79:</u>

3 Sets of 8-10 Reps Dumbbell Hammer Curls
Wt.___________________
3 Sets of 8-10 Reps Dumbbell Bent Over Triceps
Extension
Wt.___________________
3 Sets of 8-10 Reps 1 and ¼ Straight Bar (Barbell) Bicep
Curls (¼ at the top)
Wt.___________________
3 Sets of 8-10 Reps 1 ¼ Skull Crushers (¼ at the top)
Wt.___________________
3 Sets of 8-10 Reps Single Cable Bicep Curls (8-10 Reps
Each Arm)
Wt.___________________
3 Sets of 8-10 Reps Single Cable Triceps Extension (8-
10 Reps Each Arm)
Wt.___________________

3 Rounds for Time:
50 Jumping Jacks
20 Cable Machine Crunches
20 Dips
20 KB Hammer Curls
50 Flutter Kicks
Time: ___________

Cardio:
Treadmill: 10 X 1:30 Minute Sprint on Level 10-12
Speed (Sub 6-8 Minute Pace) 30 Seconds of Rest after
each set / Incline Level 8
Sets Completed: __ __ __ __ __ __ __ __ __ __

<u>Workout 80:</u>

3 Sets of 8-10 Reps Military Press
Wt.________________
3 Sets of 8-10 Reps DB Arnold Press
Wt.________________
3 Sets of 8-10 Reps Cable Front Shoulder Raise
Wt.________________
3 Sets of 8-10 Reps Cable Side Shoulder Raise
Wt.________________
3 Sets of 8-10 Reps DB Overhead Press
Wt.________________
3 Sets of 8-10 Reps Cable Overhead Press
Wt.________________

3 Rounds for Time:
50 Small Arm Circles Forward
50 Russian Twists
25 KB Swings
25 KB High Pull or Barbell High Pull
50 Reverse Crunches
50 Small Arm Circles Backward
Time: ___________

Cardio:
2 Mile Run at 6:00-8:00 Minute per mile pace – Goal is
sub 12:00 minute completion
Time: ___________
1000 Meters Rowing Machine
Time: ___________

<u>Workout 81:</u>

3 Sets of 8-10 Reps Weighted Pull Ups
Wt._______________
3 Sets of 8-10 Reps Cable Standing Lat Push-downs
Wt._______________
3 Sets of 8-10 Reps Cable Seated Rows
Wt._______________
3 Sets of 8-10 Reps Machine Back Fly
Wt._______________
3 Sets of 8-10 Reps Bent Over Dumbbell Rows
Wt._______________
3 Sets of 8-10 Reps Seated Lat Pull Down
Wt._______________

3 Rounds for Time:
20 Bent Over Dumbbell Back Fly
20 Jumping/Kipping Pull-ups
20 Push-ups
30 Cable Crunches
30 Core Twists / Russian Twists
30 Bicycle Crunches
50 Crunches
Time: ___________

Cardio:
10 Minutes on Bike at RPM +100
Distance: ___________
20 Minutes on Elliptical at HR 145-165
Distance: ___________
30 Minutes on Stair climber

<u>Workout 82:</u>

3 Sets of 8-10 Reps Barbell Front Squats
Wt.______________
3 Sets of 8-10 Reps Per Single Leg Extension
Wt.______________
3 Sets of 8-10 Reps Per Single Leg Curl
Wt.______________
3 Sets of 8-10 Reps Weighted Seated Leg Press
Wt.______________
3 Sets of 8-10 Reps Machine Calf Raise
Wt.______________
3 Sets of 8-10 Reps Bench Split Squat Per Leg
Wt.______________

3 Rounds for Time:
20 Burpees
20 Jumping Squats
20 Jumping Lunges
20 Bunny Hops (Toe Jumps)
20 Band Dirty Dogs
20 Band Donkey Kicks
50 Flutter Kicks
Time: ___________

Cardio:
2 Mile Sprint with Goal Time of 12:00 Minutes
Time: ___________
30 Minutes of Walking on Treadmill with Incline at 12
Distance: ___________

<u>Workout 83:</u>

3 Sets of 8-10 Reps Cable Bicep Curls
Wt._______________
20 Diamond Pushups
3 Sets of 8-10 Reps Cable Overhead Triceps Extension
Wt._______________
20 Diamond Pushups
3 Sets of 8-10 Reps Seated Incline Dumbbell Curls
Wt._______________
20 Diamond Pushups
3 Sets of 8-10 Reps Standing Cable Triceps Extension
Wt._______________
3 Sets of 8-10 Reps Seated Dumbbell Hammer Curls
Wt._______________

3 Rounds for Time:
30 Second Plank
30 Bicycle Crunches
30 Second Left Oblique Plank
30 Crunches
30 Second Right Oblique Plank
30 Reverse Crunches
Time: ___________

Cardio:
1.5 Mile Run at 6:00-8:00 Minute Pace Per Mile on
Treadmill Time: ___________
Bike 15 Minutes at over 100 RPM (HR 145-165)
Distance: ___________
1.5 Mile Run at 6:00-8:00 Minute Pace Per Mile on
Treadmill Time: ___________

<u>Workout 84:</u>

3 Sets of 8-10 Reps Lat Pull Down Close Grip
Wt._______________
3 Sets of 8-10 Reps Seated Military Press
Wt._______________
3 Sets of 8-10 Reps Seated Cable Row Wide Grip
Wt._______________
3 Sets of 8-10 Reps Machine Shoulder Press
Wt._______________
3 Sets of 8-10 Reps Barbell Shrugs
Wt._______________
3 Sets of 8-10 Reps Cable Machine Back Fly
Wt._______________

3 Rounds for Time:
10 Pull-Ups
20 Standing Knees-to-Elbow Cross
10 Dumbbell Overhead Press
20 Flutter Kicks
10 Pushups
20 Bicycle Crunches
Time: ___________

Cardio:
3 Mile Jog at 8:00-10:00 Min Mile Pace Per Mile (Goal
Completion Time: 24 Minutes)
Time: ___________
1 Mile Cool Down Walk
Time: ___________

Workout 85:

3 Sets of 8-10 Reps Barbell Front Squats
Wt._______________
3 Sets of 8-10 Reps Barbell Romanian Deadlifts
Wt._______________
3 Sets of 8-10 Reps Machine 1 Leg Curls
Wt._______________
3 Sets of 8-10 Reps of Machine 1 Leg Extensions
Wt._______________
3 Sets of 8-10 Reps Cable Machine Decelerated Lunges
Wt._______________
3 Sets of 8-10 Reps Kettle Bell Goblet Squat
Wt._______________
3 Sets of 8-10 Reps Machine Shrugs
Wt._______________

3 Rounds for Time:
20 Box Jumps
20 Jumping Squats
20 Jumping Lunges
20 Bunny Hops
20 Jumping Jacks
Time: ___________

Cardio:
35 Minute Treadmill Walk on Incline Level 12
Distance: ___________

<u>Workout 86:</u>

3 Sets of 8-10 Reps Close Grip Barbell Bench Press
Wt.______________
3 Sets of 8-10 Reps Incline Dumbbell Bench Press
Wt.______________
3 Sets of 8-10 Reps Decline Cable Press
Wt.______________
3 Sets of 8-10 Reps Incline Cable Press
Wt.______________
3 Sets of 8-10 Reps Cable Chest Fly
Wt.______________
3 Sets of 8-10 Reps Weighted Dips
Wt.______________

3 Rounds for Time:
20 Burpees or Up/Downs
20 Core Twists (Russian Twists)
20 Pushups
20 Bicycle Crunches
20 Jumping Jacks
Time: ___________

Cardio:
1000 Meter Rowing Machine
Time: ___________
25 Min on Elliptical maintaining HR between 145-165
Distance: ___________

<u>Workout 87:</u>

3 Sets of 8-10 Reps Barbell Preacher Curls
Wt._______________
3 Sets of 8-10 Reps Cable Triceps Extension
Wt._______________
3 Sets of 8-10 Reps Barbell Skull Crushers
Wt._______________
3 Sets of 8-10 Reps Cable Bicep Curls
Wt._______________
3 Sets of 8-10 Reps Dumbbell Hammer Curls
Wt._______________
3 Sets of 8-10 Reps Dumbbell Triceps Extension
Wt._______________

3 Rounds for Time:
20 Kettle Bell Hammer Curls
20 Kettle Bell Overhead Triceps Extension
20 Diamond Push Ups
20 Flutter Kicks
20 Bicycle Crunches
Time: ___________

Cardio:
20 Minutes Stair Climber
20 Minutes Elliptical (HR 145-165)
Distance: ___________
1000 Meter Row on Rowing Machine
Time: ___________

<u>Workout 88:</u>

3 Sets of 8-10 Reps Machine Leg Extensions
Wt.________________
3 Sets of 8-10 Reps Machine Leg Curls
Wt.________________
3 Sets of 8-10 Reps Barbell Shrugs (2 Second hold)
Wt.________________
3 Sets of 8-10 Reps 1 and ¼ Barbell Squats
Wt.________________
3 Sets of 8-10 Reps Machine Calf Raise
Wt.________________
3 Sets of 8-10 Reps Romanian Deadlifts
Wt.________________

3 Rounds for Time:
30 Air Squats
30 Second 2 Kettle Bell Farmers Carry
30 Walking Lunges
30 Second Front Plank
30 Second Side Plank (Each Side)
30 Mountain Climbers
Time: ____________

Cardio:
20 Minutes Stair Climber
20 Minutes Walking at Incline 10-12 on Treadmill
Distance: ____________

<u>Workout 89:</u>

3 Sets of 8-10 Reps Barbell Hang Clean
Wt.________________
3 Sets of 8-10 Reps Dumbbell Arnold Press
Wt.________________
3 Sets of 8-10 Reps Seated Lateral Dumbbell Raise
Wt.________________
3 Sets of 8-10 Reps Barbell Bent over Rows
Wt.________________
3 Sets of 8-10 Reps Machine Lat Pull Down Wide Grip
Wt.________________
3 Sets of 8-10 Reps Cable Face Pulls
Wt.________________
3 Sets of 8-10 Reps Cable Back Fly
Wt.________________

3 Rounds for Time:
10 Pull Ups
20 Push Ups
30 V-Ups
40 Jumping Jacks
50 Crunches
Time: ___________

Cardio:
2000 Meter Rowing Machine Row (Goal= Under 20
Minutes) Time: ___________
5 X ¼ Mile Sprints (Goal= Under 2 Minutes Per ¼ Mile)
45 Second Rest in between sets
Sets Completed: __ __ __ __ __

<u>Workout 90:</u>

3 Sets of 8-10 Reps Reverse Grip Barbell Bench Press
Wt._______________
3 Sets of 8-10 Reps Close Grip Barbell Bench Press
Wt._______________
3 Sets of 8-10 Reps Seated Dumbbell Curls
Wt._______________
3 Sets of 8-10 Reps Seated Dumbbell Overhead Triceps Extension
Wt._______________
3 Sets of 8-10 Reps Cable Fly
Wt._______________
3 Sets of 8-10 Reps Cable Decline Chest Press
Wt._______________
3 Sets of 8-10 Reps Cable Incline Chest Press
Wt._______________

3 Rounds for Time:
30 Push Ups
30 Russian Twists (Core Twists)
30 Jumping Jacks
30 Flutter Kicks
30 Mountain Climbers
Time: ___________

Cardio:
500 Meter Row
Time: ___________
25 Burpees
2 Mile Jog at 8:00-10:00 Minute Per Mile Pace
Time: ___________

<u>Workout 91:</u>

3 Sets of 8-10 Reps Machine Leg Extension (2 Sec Hold at Top)
Wt.______________
3 Sets of 8-10 Reps Machine Leg Curls (2 Sec Hold at Top)
Wt.______________
3 Sets of 8-10 Reps Machine Leg Press
Wt.______________
3 Sets of 8-10 Reps Barbell 1 and ¼ Squats
Wt.______________
3 Sets of 8-10 Reps Barbell Calf Raise
Wt.______________
3 Sets of 8-10 Reps Machine Calf Raise
Wt.______________
3 Sets of 8-10 Reps Barbell Lunges
Wt.______________

3 Rounds for Time:
20 Dumbbell Box Step Ups
20 Walking Lunges (10 Per Leg)
20 Dumbbell Thrusters
20 V-Ups
20 Russian Twists / Core Twists
Time: __________

Cardio:
5 Mile Treadmill Run on Incline 8 (Goal= Under 45 Minutes or Sub 8:00 Minute Mile Pace Per Mile)
Time: __________

<u>Workout 92:</u>

3 Sets of 8-10 Reps Barbell Curls
Wt._________________
3 Sets of 8-10 Reps Skull Crushers
Wt._________________
3 Sets of 8-10 Reps Cable Rope Bicep Curls
Wt._______________
3 Sets of 8-10 Reps Cable Rope Triceps Extensions
Wt._______________
3 Sets of 8-10 Reps Dumbbell Hammer Curls
Wt._______________
3 Sets of 8-10 Reps Bent Over Dumbbell Triceps
Extension
Wt._______________

3 Rounds for Time:
20 Dips
20 Flutter Kicks
20 Close Grip Push Ups (Diamond)
20 Hanging Knee Raise
20 Russian Twists
Time: ___________

Cardio:
10 X ¼ Mile Sprints (Goal= Under 2 Minutes Per ¼
Mile) 45 Second Rest in between sets
Sets Completed: __ __ __ __ __ __ __ __ __ __
1 Mile Sprint (Goal=6:00 Minute Mile)
Time: ___________

<u>Workout 93:</u>

3 Sets of 8-10 Reps Dumbbell Standing Front Raise
Wt.______________
3 Sets of 8-10 Reps Dumbbell Standing Lateral Raise
Wt.______________
3 Sets of 8-10 Reps Seated Dumbbell Overhead Arnold Press
Wt.______________
3 Sets of 8-10 Reps Barbell Shrugs
Wt.______________
3 Sets of 8-10 Reps Cable High Pull
Wt.______________
3 Sets of 8-10 Reps Cable Face Pulls
Wt.______________

3 Rounds for Time:
30 Overhead Air Press
30 Large Arm Circles Forward
30 Large Arm Circles Backward
30 Russian Twists (Core Twists)
30 Second Plank
Time: __________

Cardio:
20 Minutes Stair Climber Machine
20 Minutes on Elliptical (145-165 HR)
Distance: __________

<u>Workout 94:</u>

3 Sets of 8-10 Reps Cable Machine Decelerating Lunges
(per leg)
Wt._______________
3 Sets of 8-10 Reps Barbell Romanian Deadlifts
Wt._______________
3 Sets of 8-10 Reps Leg Extension (Hold at top 2 sec)
Wt._______________
3 Sets of 8-10 Reps Machine Leg Curls (Hold 2 sec)
Wt._______________
3 Sets of 8-10 Reps Machine Leg Press (4 Count Down)
Wt._______________
3 Sets of 8-10 Reps Machine Calf Raise (Hold 2 sec)
Wt._______________
3 Sets of 8-10 Reps Barbell Split Squats (Per leg)
Wt._______________

3 Rounds for Time:
20 Dumbbell Box Step Ups
20 Dumbbell Standing Calf Raise
20 Mountain Climbers
20 Reverse Crunches
20 Jumping Jacks
Time: ___________

Cardio:
10 X 2:00 minute Sprint at 6:00-8:00 Min. Mile Pace
(Incline Level 8-10)
Sets Completed: __ __ __ __ __ __ __ __ __ __
10 Minutes Elliptical (HR 145-165)
Distance: _________

Workout 95

3 Sets of 8-10 Reps Cable Lat Pull Downs
Wt.________________
3 Sets of 8-10 Reps Bent Over Dumbbell Rows
Wt.________________
3 Sets of 8-10 Reps Seated Cable Machine Rows
Wt.________________
3 Sets of 8-10 Reps Cable Machine Back Fly
Wt.________________
3 Sets of 8-10 Reps Bent Over Barbell Rows
Wt.________________
3 Sets of 8-10 Reps Barbell Deadlifts
Wt.________________

3 Rounds for Time:
20 Kipping Pull Ups
500-meter Rowing Machine Row
20 Reverse Flutter Kicks
20 Flutter Kicks
20 Push Ups
Time: __________

Cardio:
6 X ¼ Mile Sprint (Goal= Under 2:00 Minutes per Sprint) Sets Completed: __ __ __ __ __ __
4 X ½ Mile Sprint (Goal= Under 3:30 Minutes Per Sprint) Sets Completed: __ __ __ __
10 Minutes on Bicycle RPM 100+
Distance: __________

<u>Workout 96</u>

3 Sets of 8-10 Reps Cable Triceps Extension
Wt._____________
3 Sets of 8-10 Reps Cable Straight Bar Bicep Curls
Wt._____________
3 Sets of 8-10 Reps Bench Press
Wt._____________
3 Sets of 8-10 Reps Cable Decline Press
Wt._____________
3 Sets of 8-10 Reps Cable Incline Press
Wt._____________
3 Sets of 8-10 Reps Single Cable Bicep Curl
Wt._____________
3 Sets of 8-10 Reps Single Cable Triceps Extension
Wt._____________

3 Rounds for Time:
20 Dips
20 Dumbbell Hammer Curls (10 Each Arm)
20 Bent Over Dumbbell Triceps Extension (10 Each Arm)
20 Push Ups
20 Knee Raises
20 Decline Push Ups
Time: __________

Cardio:
1.5 Mile Run (Goal of Under 10 Minutes)
Time: __________
1.5 Mile Treadmill Walk on Incline Level 12
Distance: __________

<u>Workout 97</u>

3 Sets of 8-10 Reps Barbell Squats
Wt._______________
3 Sets of 8-10 Reps Leg Extension (2 Second Hold)
Wt._______________
3 Sets of 8-10 Reps Leg Curls (2 Second Hold)
Wt._____________
3 Sets of 8-10 Reps Barbell Calf Raise
Wt._______________
3 Sets of 8-10 Reps Romanian Deadlifts
Wt._______________
3 Sets of 8-10 Reps Cable Lunges Decelerating
Wt._______________

3 Rounds for Time:
20 Bunny Hops
20 Band Resistance Donkey Kicks
20 Band Resistance Dirty Dogs
20 Box Jumps (Step Ups for Scale)
20 Reverse Crunches
20 Russian Twists
20 Air Squats
Time: __________

Cardio:
5 X 1:00 Minute Sprints (6:00 Minute Mile Pace on
Treadmill) 30 Sec Rest In between Sprints
Sets Completed: __ __ __ __ __
1 Mile Jog (8:00-10:00 Minute Mile Pace)
Time: __________
20 Minutes Stair Climber Machine

Workout 98

3 Sets of 8-10 Reps Seated Cable Rows
Wt._________________
3 Sets of 8-10 Reps Standing Cable Lat Push Down
Wt._________________
3 Sets of 8-10 Reps Cable Face Pulls
Wt._________________
3 Sets of 8-10 Reps Cable Overhead Press
Wt._________________
3 Sets of 8-10 Reps Reverse Grip Lat Pull Down
Wt._________________
3 Sets of 8-10 Reps Cable Straight Bar High Pulls
Wt._________________

3 Rounds for Time:
10 Pull Ups
20 Dumbbell Back Fly
20 Bent Over Barbell Rows
20 Kettlebell Swings
20 Dumbbell Front Raise
50 Crunches
Time: ___________

Cardio:
15 Minutes on the Elliptical maintaining HR at 145-165
Distance: __________
5 Mile Bike Ride
Time: ___________
1000 Meter Row on Rowing Machine
Time: ___________

<u>Workout 99:</u>

3 Sets of 8-10 Reps Decline Cable Chest Press
Wt.________________
3 Sets of 8-10 Reps Incline Cable Chest Press
Wt.________________
3 Sets of 8-10 Reps Cable Fly
Wt.________________
3 Sets of 8-10 Reps Cable Triceps Extensions
Wt.________________
3 Sets of 8-10 Reps Hammer Rope Cable Curls
Wt.________________
3 Sets of 8-10 Reps Straight Bar Cable Triceps
Extensions Wt.________________
3 Sets of 8-10 Reps Straight Bar Cable Biceps Curl
Wt.________________

3 Rounds for Time:
30 Push Ups
30 Dips
30 Russian Twists
30 Bicycle Crunches
30 Jumping Jacks
30 Kettlebell Hammer Curls
30 Burpees
Time: __________

Cardio:
5 Mile Run at 6:00-8:00 Minute Per Mile Pace
Time: __________

<u>Workout 100:</u>

3 Sets of 8-10 Reps Barbell Front Squats
Wt.______________
3 Sets of 8-10 Reps Barbell Split Squats
Wt.______________
3 Sets of 8-10 Reps Machine Leg Extensions
Wt.______________
3 Sets of 8-10 Reps Machine Leg Curls
Wt.______________
3 Sets of 8-10 Reps Barbell Deadlifts
Wt.______________
3 Sets of 8-10 Reps Cable Lunges
Wt.______________
3 Sets of 8-10 Reps Machine Leg Press
Wt.______________

3 Rounds for Time:
20 Jump Squats
20 Jumping Lunges
20 Hanging Knee Raises
20 Russian Twists
20 Bunny Hops
20 Jumping Jacks
20 Mountain Climbers
Time: ___________

Cardio:
5000 Meter Row on Rowing Machine
Time: ___________
2 Mile Treadmill Walk on Incline Level 12
Time: ___________